Table of Contents

5 Foods That Can Help Endometriosis (and 6 to Avoid) 2

6 types of food to avoid 10

How can you get pregnant with endometriosis-related infertility? 16

What's the success rate of getting pregnant with endo? 19

How to naturally improve your conception chances 21

How will endometriosis affect your pregnancy? 22

Will your kids also have endometriosis? 24

7-day meal plan for managing painful endometriosis symptoms 25

Recipes for Endometriosis 33

5 Foods That Can Help Endometriosis (and 6 to Avoid)

1. Salmon and other sources of omega-3 fatty acids

What we know about omega-3s: They play a big role in helping our bodies fight pain and inflammation, which can be especially helpful for those dealing with endometriosis.

Omega-3s also have the most scientific support of reducing the risk of developing endometriosis in the first place.

A study of 74,708 women found that patients who ate lots of omega-3s had a lower risk of endometriosis. In another study, women who ate the most salmon (and other foods rich in omega-3s) were 22 percent less likely to develop it.

If you've had your fill of salmon, try munching on mackerel, sardines, anchovies, or oysters, which are all great sources of the helpful fatty acids.

Not a fish fan? Reach for flax seeds, chia seeds, and walnuts to get your omega-3 fix.

When all else fails, turn to fish oil supplements. In a preliminary mouse study, fish oil supplements lead to a reduction of endometrial adhesions. Although, this is a very early study and it's hard to say whether the same would be true for humans.

Still, omega-3s have all kinds of health benefits, and if you'd rather not go to town on nuts and fish, a supplement might be a good option.

2. Leafy greens and whole fruits

What healthy diet list would be complete without a mention of fruits and vegetables? Both are good sources of fiber, which can lower estrogen levels and, ergo, help manage endo symptoms.

Unsurprisingly, green vegetables are an ideal place to start.

Multiple studies found that eating lots of green veggies decreases your risk of the disorder. So things like spinach, kale, Swiss chard, and arugula are great options to add to your diet.

Though leafy greens came out on top in most studies, some found that vegetable intake made no difference in the occurrence of endometriosis.

And then there's fruits. As you recall from just about every lesson in grade school, whole fruits are full of vitamins, minerals, and nutrients that do the body good.

Even better, they're loaded with antioxidants, which research suggests can reduce chronic pelvic pain in women with endometriosis.

And while we know added sugars can trigger inflammation, the naturally occurring fructose in whole fruits is A-OK. Just don't confuse a pint of raspberry ice cream for a pint of actual raspberries.

3. Oats, cherries, and almonds, oh my!

No, these aren't the ingredients for a homemade granola bar — though, it's not a bad idea if you need some meal prep inspo. They're actually all foods that are high in melatonin. Opt for tart cherries over sweet varieties.

Other than being an important sleep aid, one study found that melatonin significantly reduced endometriosis pain. The study noted that 10 mg of melatonin per day helped participants manage pain levels.

If oatmeal isn't your favorite, you can always reach for a supplement. Just be sure to check with your doctor before making any major diet changes.

4. Low-FODMAP foods

"Quit eating so many FODMAPs!" is probably not something your mom said at the dinner table. But there is some evidence that a low-FODMAP diet could help.

So, what does that mean? The low-FODMAP (fermentable oligo-, di-, mono-saccharides, and polyols) diet was developed for people with IBS to reduce symptoms of intestinal discomfort.

With this diet you avoid foods like: wheat, rye, legumes, garlic, onions, milk, yogurt, soft cheese, honey, low calorie sweeteners, and a variety of fruits.

It's a lot to give up, so it's worth noting that studies have shown that only people with IBS and endometriosis were helped by the Low-FODMAP diet.

5. Green tea

Research suggests that green tea's cancer-fighting secret ingredient EGCG can also help put endometriosis in its place.

EGCG has been found to shrink tumor cells, which is why green tea is recommended as a drink for cancer patients. Similarly, one 2008 study found that EGCG could prevent new endometriotic lesions from forming.

While we're all for having a daily tea party complete with finger sandwiches and scones, you can always turn to an EGCG supplement for relief (providing you get the OK from your doc!).

Here are a few other supplements with promising science you can check out:

- antioxidant supplements (shop here)
- soy supplements (shop here)
- turmeric supplements (shop here)

1. **Trans fats**

   Just like omega-3s have the most scientific support for reducing the risk of developing endometriosis, trans fats are on the opposite side of the coin.

   In general, trans fats lead to greater inflammation which can add to the pain and discomfort of endometriosis. Eating high levels of trans fats can also increase your risk of developing the disorder by up to 48 percent!

   As much as we love them, try to avoid foods like vegetable shortening, fried fast food, canned frosting, and non-dairy coffee creamer.

2. **Gluten**

Though "gluten-free" has become the latest outrage of middle-aged comedians, there's some proof that a gluten-free diet can help symptoms of endometriosis.

In a 2012 study from Tor Vergata University, 75 percent of the patients on a gluten-free diet had a noticeable reduction in pain. It's good to note that this is only one study and needs more proof before it's scientifically verified.

If you'd like to try a gluten-free diet to decrease pain and inflammation, it's best to go with naturally gluten-free foods like vegetables and lean meats.

Gluten-free versions of popular carbs — like bread, pasta, and baked goods — are often refined and full of extra fat and sugar to make up for the lack of gluten.

3. **Red meat**

Bacon lovers, don't shoot the messenger. A 2004 study from the University of Milano found that red meat and ham significantly increased the likelihood of endometriosis.

Before you ditch your Cheeseburger Fridays though, it's only fair to mention that there are more recent studies that have found no link at all between red meat and endometriosis.

While eating a lot of saturated fat via red meat may generally not be the best thing to do, that doesn't mean you can't ever touch a steak. Instead, try to limit your servings of red meat to once or twice per week.

4. **Coffee and alcohol (maybe)**

Coffee and alcohol would seem to be bad for endometriosis since coffee has been found to increase an estrogen protein in the body, and increased estrogen may be linked to causing endometriosis.

Some studies found increased alcohol consumption led to an increased likelihood of getting the disorder, while other studies found no link between alcohol and endometriosis.

Even more confusing, coffee and alcohol can have both inflammatory and anti-inflammatory properties, which means you might have to do some experimenting to find what works for you.

Generally, consuming either in moderation shouldn't send your body into an inflamed tailspin, but it's always best to check with your doctor.

5. **Dairy (kinda)**

Another head scratcher, here. Most studies recommend avoiding dairy — especially milk, yogurt, and cheese — to keep endometriosis symptoms in check.

However, there is some research that links low-fat dairy consumption with reduced risk of developing endometriosis, and suggests dairy has anti-inflammatory properties.

Ultimately, more research is needed and this might be a case where personal experimentation or a consultation with your doc is the way to go.

How can you get pregnant with endometriosis-related infertility?

If you've been knocking boots for 6 months to a year and haven't gotten your eggo preggo, surgical options and/or fertility treatments are likely to be your next step.

Your doctor or fertility specialist might suggest the following treatments:

- Conservative surgery. A doctor can surgically remove bits of endometrial tissue while protecting the function of your reproductive organs.
- Freezing your eggs. Because endo can reduce the number of viable eggs in your ovaries, you may want to preserve some for pregnancy in the future.

- Hysterosalpingogram. A doctor will inject dye into your uterus and take X-rays to see if your fallopian tubes are open.

- Medication. Fertility drugs like clomiphene citrate can induce ovulation or increase the number of eggs you produce at one time, increasing your chances of conception.

- Ultrasound. By scanning your ovaries every few days, a fertility specialist can tell how your eggs are developing and the best time to try to conceive.

- Intrauterine insemination (IUI). This procedure involves placing semen directly in your uterus close to ovulation to increase the odds of fertilization.

- In vitro fertilization (IVF). After you receive drugs to stimulate your ovaries, a healthcare pro will remove your eggs and fertilize them in a lab. Successfully fertilized eggs will then be implanted in your uterus.

Ready to roll the dice on pregnancy? There are a few different ways to look at how endometriosis will affect your chances of getting pregnant.

According to a 2014 review, 2 to 10 percent of couples dealing with endo will have children in their lifetime, compared with 15 to 20 percent for fertile folks.

For those who have endometriosis and don't have surgery, studies estimate that pregnancy rates are about 33 percent with moderate endo and 0 percent with severe endo. But having surgery may increase your odds.

Studies suggest that laparoscopic surgery to treat moderate endometriosis increases pregnancy rates to 57 to 69 percent. For people with severe endometriosis, the chance goes up to 52 to 68 percent after surgery.

IVF may improve those odds even further, but it's not a guarantee. In a 2005 study, 56 percent of women with moderate to severe endometriosis got pregnant after 1 to 4 IVF treatments, and about 40 percent actually gave birth. But it's been tough for researchers to determine exact percentages.

How to naturally improve your conception chances

Beyond medical treatments, improving your fertility with endometriosis is basically the same as improving fertility in general.

Here are some tips to boost your well-being and chances of getting pregnant:

- Eat a varied diet to hit all your essential nutrients.
- Track your cycle to plan sex around ovulation.
- Keep your body moving with daily exercise.
- Take steps to reduce stress (hello, yoga and meditation!).
- Get enough sleep.

Having endometriosis doesn't guarantee that you'll have pregnancy complications. But complications are possible, so your doctor may recommend extra monitoring during your pregnancy.

A 2017 study of more than 19,000 births found that people with endometriosis had a higher risk of severe high blood pressure, hemorrhage, problems with the placenta, and premature broken waters.

The babies in the study had an increased risk of being born before 28 weeks' gestation, small size for gestational age, congenital malformations, and death.

Having endometrial surgery before pregnancy also comes with increased risks. One study found that people who had surgery to treat endometriosis were more likely to have placenta previa, a condition in which the placenta blocks the cervix, making vaginal delivery risky and warranting a cesarean delivery.

According to a 2018 research review, endometriosis is also associated with higher risk of gestational diabetes, cesarean delivery, and neonatal intensive care unit admission for the baby.

Will your kids also have endometriosis?

There does seem to be hereditary link to endometriosis.

Studies of people with confirmed endometriosis have shown "familial clustering." It's estimated that siblings, parents, and children of people with endometriosis are 5 to 7 times more likely to have endo than people who don't have a first-degree relative with the condition.

So if you give birth to a female kiddo (and your mom, sis, or aunt also has endo), it *is* possible your kid could have it too.

Living a healthy lifestyle, taking pain-relief medication like NSAIDs, or in some cases, hormone therapy, and implementing an anti-inflammatory diet, also known as the "endometriosis diet," may relieve endometriosis-related pain and reduce symptoms — though more research is needed to determine how effective diet, alone, can be.

"The endometriosis diet involves limiting certain foods that can exacerbate inflammation and pain," says Tara Scott, MD, and founder of Revitalize Medical Group.

Between 3.8% and 37% of individuals with endometriosis are affected by bowel endometriosis or intestinal endometriosis. "So, by cleaning up your diet, you can clean up your gut," Scott says.

Here are common foods to eat and avoid as well as a 7-day meal plan that may help manage endometriosis-related symptoms.

Monday

Stir Fry

- Breakfast: Mixed vegetable stir fry with organic firm tofu and ½ cup quinoa, a slice of melon, and one cup of an English breakfast tea (~444 calories)
- Lunch: Half an avocado with hummus, and one cup of green tea (~264 calories)
- Dinner: One bowl of chicken soup with vegetables with one cup of basmati rice with organic cassava tortillas, a baked apple with walnuts and raisins and coconut whipped

cream, and one cup of camomile tea (~896 calories)

- Total for the day: ~1,604 calories

Tuesday

Chili

- Warm up for dinner with a bowl of vegetarian chili. Annabelle Breakey/Getty Images
- Breakfast: One large bowl of millet with nuts, seeds, dates, one cup of organic soy milk, a sliced pear, and one cup of Earl Gray tea (~508 calories)
- Lunch: One hard-boiled egg and a handful of walnuts, mixed greens, and one cup of green tea (~285 calories)
- Dinner: One bowl of vegetarian chili, organic corn tortillas, cashew yogurt, mixed green

salad with balsamic dressing, a sliced orange, and one cup of hibiscus tea (~1,081 calories)

- Total for the day: ~1,874 calories

Wednesday (modified fast day)

Avocado

- Breakfast: Five macadamia nuts (~93 calories)
- Lunch: One-fourth of an avocado (~80 calories)
- Dinner: Six walnut halves and unlimited herbal tea (~78 calories)
- Total for the day: ~251 calories

Thursday

Nuts

- Mixed nuts are a good snack, just be sure to not overdo it since they're also high in calories. Peter Dazeley/Getty Images

- Breakfast: Scrambled eggs with vegetables stir fry, organic corn tortillas, ½ of a grapefruit, and one cup of black tea (~387 calories)

- Lunch: One baked sweet potato, edamame, mixed raw nuts, and one cup of green tea (~334 calories)

- Dinner: Beyond burger meatballs, gluten-free pasta, tomato sauce, tossed salad, one gluten-free bread slice, sautéed bananas, and one cup of cinnamon tea (~870 calories)

- Total for the day: ~1,592 calories

Friday

Roasted Vegetables

- Breakfast: One large bowl of buckwheat, varied nuts and seeds, organic almond slivers, sliced mango, organic decaf coffee, and a splash of almond milk (~861 calories)
- Lunch: Small green salad with olives and seeds in olive oil, and one cup of green tea (~281 calories)
- Dinner: Organic wild salmon (baked), broccoli, carrots, beets, roasted potatoes, sautéed pear, and one cup of ginger tea (~843 calories)
- Total for the day: ~1,985 calories

Saturday (modified fast day)

Salad

- Add a refreshing green salad to your dinner. BURCU ATALAY TANKUT/Getty Images
- Breakfast: Six walnut halves and one cup of green tea (~80 calories)
- Lunch: One-fourth of an avocado and one cup of spearmint tea (~80 calories)
- Dinner: Small green salad with olive oil (~140 calories)
- Total for the day: ~300 calories

Sunday

Pancakes

- Breakfast: Gluten-free pancakes with fresh berries, cashew or coconut yogurt, organic decaf coffee, and organic soy milk, fresh orange slices (~636 calories)

- Lunch: Celery and apple slices with almond butter (~162 calories)

- Dinner: Tossed salad and balsamic dressing, grilled prawns on basmati rice, ratatouille, sliced papaya, mango, and one cup of rooibos tea (~728 calories)

1. **Anti-Inflammatory Breakfast Recipes**

   Ingredients

   - approximately 2 inches of fresh raw ginger, peeled and finely sliced

   - 1 1/2 – 2 cups of water

   - a squeeze of fresh lemon juice (optional)

   - optional add-ins: a pinch of turmeric and/or cinnamon, natural sweetener

   Instructions

   Infusion Method for Ginger Tea

   - Boil water in a kettle, let it settle then pour the just-boiled water into a mug with the peeled and sliced ginger and let sit for 5-10 minutes, or to taste. Strain the ginger pieces out. Add optional lemon, optional sweetener such as raw honey, whole leaf stevia powder or stevia extract, brown rice syrup, agave nectar or pure maple syrup and a pinch of turmeric.

Decoction Method for Ginger Tea

- Bring the ginger and water to a light boil stovetop and let boil for 15-10 minutes, covered. The longer it simmers, the stronger it will be.
- Remove from heat and add lemon, optional sweetener and a pinch of turmeric if you'd like.

2. **Superfoods Detox Smoothie**

Ingredients

- 2 cups freshly squeezed orange juice, or equal quantity peeled and pitted oranges
- 1 unpeeled, pitted apple
- 1 ripe banana

- 3 tablespoons goji berries

- 1 teaspoon turmeric

- A pinch of pepper

- 1 teaspoon cinnamon

- 2 tablespoons tahini (you can up this to 4 tablespoons or even replace with almond butter)

- 3 brazil nuts

- 2 teaspoons fresh grated ginger

- 3 teaspoons chia seeds

Instructions

- Blend all ingredients until smooth.

- Drink!

3. **Green Smoothie**

Ingredients

- 2 cups spinach

- 2 cups water

- 1 cup mango

- 1 cup pineapple

- 2 bananas Use at least one frozen fruit to chill your smoothie. We often use frozen mangos and bananas our green smoothies.

Instructions

- Tightly pack 2 cups of leafy greens in a measuring cup and then toss into blender.

- Add water and blend together until all leafy chunks are gone.

- Add mango, pineapple and bananas and blend again until smooth.

- Pour into a mason jar (or cute cup of your choice).

- Gulp or sip like a rawkstar!

4. **Anti-Inflammatory Healing Bowl with Sweet Potatoes, Turmeric and Kale**

Equipment

- Tools
- Large bowl
- Baking sheet
- Skillet

Ingredients

- 2 sweet potatoes, cubed (roughly 3 cups cubed)
- 2 T coconut oil, divided
- 1 red bell pepper, diced
- 1 red onion, diced
- 3 garlic cloves, minced
- 1 t ground turmeric
- ½ t pepper
- 2 cups chopped kale, ribs removed

- Salt to taste

- 2 eggs

- 1 avocado, sliced lengthwise

Instructions

- Preheat the oven to 400°F.

- Toss the cubed sweet potatoes in one tablespoon of coconut oil in a large bowl. Coat evenly before transferring to a baking sheet.

- Roast the sweet potatoes for at least 30 minutes, until they are fully cooked and golden brown on the edges. Make sure to flip them over halfway through.

- While the sweet potatoes roast, sauté the diced bell peppers and red onion with the remaining 1 tablespoon of coconut oil in a large skillet, until the vegetables are tender.

- Add the minced garlic, ground turmeric, and pepper, mixing well for about 20 seconds.

- Add the chopped kale and cook until wilted. Add salt to taste, then set aside.
- Wipe the skillet (careful, it may be hot) and cook two sunny-side-up eggs. Sprinkle with salt and pepper.
- Serve the roasted sweet potatoes in a large bowl layered with the sautéed vegetables, sunny-side-up eggs, and sliced avocado.

5. **Paleo Avocado Sweet Potato Toast Recipe**

Ingredients

- 2 large sweet potatoes, ends removed and sliced lengthwise into ¼-inch (0.65 cm) thick slices
- Salt, to taste
- 2 large avocados, mashed
- 1/4 cup (60 ml) Paleo pizza sauce or tomato sauce

Instructions

- Preheat oven to 400 F (200 C).

- To make the sweet potato toast, sprinkle the toast with salt and place on a greased rimmed baking sheet.

- Bake for 30 minutes, flipping in the middle. (Alternatively, toast the slices without the avocado oil in a toaster on high for 5 minutes per slice.)

- Spread mashed avocado on each slice and top with a dash of pizza sauce.

6. **Sweet potato and walnut salad**

Ingredients

- 1kg gold sweet potato, cut crossways into 1cm-thick slices

- 2 tbsp olive oil

- 2 garlic cloves, thinly sliced

- 1/2 cup (50g) walnuts

- 120g pkt Coles Superfood Leaf Blend

- 2 x 250g pkts cooked baby beetroot, quartered

- 1/4 cup (60ml) balsamic dressing

Directions

- reheat oven to 200C. Combine sweet potato, oil and garlic in a roasting pan. Roast for 40 mins or until sweet potato is tender.

- Add walnuts and cook for a further 5 mins or until walnuts are toasted. Set aside for 20 mins to cool.

- Arrange the sweet potato mixture, salad leaves and beetroot on a serving platter. Drizzle with dressing. Season.

7. **Asian Chicken Lettuce Wraps (Better Than Pf Chang's!)**

INGREDIENTS

- 2 tbsp chopped garlic
- 1 large shallot, chopped
- 1.5 tbsp chopped ginger, about 3 thin slices
- ⅔ cup chopped carrots, about 1 medium size carrot
- ⅔ cup chopped celery
- 5-6 whole water chestnuts, chopped, optional
- ½ lb. raw shrimp, peeled, devined, and diced. See notes.
- 2 tbsp Avocado oil
- ½ lb. ground chicken breast, (see notes)
- ¼ tsp coarse salt, or to taste
- ⅛ tsp white pepper

Sauce:

- 3 tbsp almond butter
- 2 tbsp coconut aminos
- 2 tsp hot pepper sauce, optional
- 3-4 tbsp apple juice , or water

Serve and garnish:

- 1-2 heads Butter lettuce
- 3 tbsp Toasted almond or cashew nuts, chopped
- 1 bulb scallion, chopped

Instructions

- Prepare ingredients from garlic to chestnuts. If use shrimp, dice it to bite size. Prepare the sauce in one bowl. Set them aside ready to use.
- In a well-heated large skillet or wok, add 2 tbsp oil. Saute garlic, shallot, and ginger over

medium high heat with a pinch of salt until fragrant, about 10 seconds.

- Add ground chicken. Season with salt and pepper. Saute until the meat is cooked through, about 2-3 minutes. Then lower the heat to medium, saute for 2 additional minutes. Your skillet should not be wet and watery or the dish will be less tasty.

- Turn the heat up to medium-high, add carrots and celery. Season with a pinch of salt. Saute for 1 minute. Add chestnuts and shrimp, if using. Saute for another 1 minute.

- Add 2 tbsp sauce and stir-fry for coat it all over, about 10 seconds. Keep the sauce minimal so the texture remains crunchy and not soggy. Taste and make seasoning adjustments to your liking. Off heat.

- To serve, place the lettuce wraps over a large serving tray/plate. Load each lettuce cup with several tablespoons of the mixture into the center. Garnish with scallions and nuts. Serve the extra sauce on the side. Serve in room temperature.

8. Taco Chicken Salad

Ingredients

- 3–4 cups cooked chicken, diced
- 1/2 cup mayo, or to taste
- 1/2 green pepper, diced
- 1/2 red pepper, diced
- 1/2 cup red onion, diced
- 1/2 medium tomato, diced
- 1/2 cup chopped cilantro
- 1 tablespoon chili powder
- 1/2 tablespoon garlic powder
- 1/4 tablespoon paprika
- 1/2 teaspoon cumin

- 1/4 teaspoon cayenne
- 1/4 teaspoon chipotle powder
- Juice of 1/2 lime

Instructions

- In a large bowl, mix mayo with the spices first to evenly combine
- Add in chicken and vegetables, mix well to evenly coat with seasoned mayo
- Squeeze lime juice over chicken salad and mix again to combine
- Top with any additional garnishes (more cilantro, diced green onion)
- Store in the refrigerator in an airtight container

9. **Paleo Italian Salad Recipe**

Ingredients

Oregano Vinaigrette

- 1/2 cup avocado oil or extra virgin olive oil

- 2 tablespoons mayonnaise

- 3 tablespoons red wine vinegar

- 2 tablespoons garlic cloves minced

- 1/4-1/2 teaspoons salt

- 1/4 teaspoon black pepper

- 2 teaspoons Italian seasoning

For Salad:

- 1 head radicchio , chopped, about 4 cups

- 1 head romaine lettuce , stem cut off and sliced thin

- 1/4 cup sliced red onion

- 1/2 cup grape tomatoes , halved

- 1/4 cup kalamata olives , pitted and sliced

- 1/4 cup black olives , pitted and sliced

- 1/2-3/4 cup Italian dry salami , sliced

- 1/4 cup sun-dried tomatoes , sliced

- 2/3 cup Mezzetta Peperoncini , stemmed, deseeded and sliced

- 2-4 whole medium-boiled eggs , diced

- 1/4 cup chopped marinated artichoke hearts

- 1/4 cup chopped roasted garlic cloves

Instructions

Make Dressing

- Combine all ingredients in a food processor and blend until very smooth. Or combine all ingredients in a medium bowl and whisk until emulsified and well-blended.

Make Salad

- In a large bowl, combine all ingredients. Pour salad dressing over, a little at a time, and toss with tongs until well coated. Serve immediately.

10. ONE POT LEMON CHICKEN AND ASPARAGUS

Ingredients

- 2 tbsp olive oil

- 4 chicken breasts

- 1 lemon, sliced into thin rounds

- 4 cloves garlic

- 1 tsp oregano

- 1 bunch of asparagus, woody parts trimmed and then cut into 1" strips

- salt and pepper, to taste

Instructions

- Preheat oven to 400 degrees.

- Heat cast iron pan on stove on medium high.

- Add olive oil to hot pan and heat until shimmery.

- Add chicken to pan and brown.

- Remove from stove and add lemon, garlic and oregano into pan.

- Cook in oven until chicken reaches 155 degrees internally, about 25 minutes.

- Add asparagus to pan.

- Continue to heat until asparagus is soft and chicken has reached internal temperature of 175 degrees, about another 20 minutes.

- Serve immediately with salad, rice, or vegetables.

11. Keto Thai Red Beef Curry

Ingredients:

- 2 - 2 1/2 pounds pastured chuck steak, cubed

- 2 tablespoons Thai red curry paste with no added preservatives or sugar

- 1/4 cup beef bone broth, warmed

- 1 teaspoon turmeric powder

- One 14-ounce can coconut cream (not coconut milk; BPA-free)

- 1 fresh kaffir lime leaf (or zest and juice from 1/2 lime)

- 3/4 tsp salt (if curry paste is salt-free)

Instructions:

- Preheat the oven to 210 degrees.

- In a large bowl, whisk curry paste with turmeric, salt and bone broth until combined. If using lime juice and zest instead of kaffir lime leaf, add to the mixture.

- Add meat and coconut cream and stir through until the meat is evenly coated.

- Pour the mixture into an ovenproof dish and wedge the kaffir lime leaf (if using) into the meat. Place the lid on top and bake for 2 hours.

- After 2 hours, give the mix a good stir and place it back in the oven (without the lid) and cook for another 1-1.5 hours.

- If the meat is tender and almost falling apart, remove the dish from the oven. If not, continue cooking for another 40 minutes or until the meat is tender.

- When cooked, carefully remove all the meat pieces from the dish and place them into a bowl. Set aside.

- Keep the juices in the oven proof dish and place it back into the oven. Turn the heat up to 320 degrees and keep cooking the liquid for another 40 minutes, or until the sauce has reduced by half.

- Remove dish from the oven and carefully return meat to the sauce.

- Serve warm with zoodles, cauliflower rice, or steamed greens.

12. JALAPEÑO TURKEY BURGERS!

Ingredients

- 1 pound ground turkey, I prefer 85% lean, it has more fat which makes for a better burger! If your ground turkey has excess liquid, be sure to set on paper towels to remove the juices.
- 1/2-3/4 of one jalapeño pepper, minced (I like it hot so I use 3/4)
- 1 medium size shallot, peeled and minced
- zest of one lime
- 2 Tablespoons chopped cilantro
- 1 teaspoon paprika
- 1 teaspoon cumin
- 1/2 a teaspoon sea salt
- 1/2 teaspoon black pepper
- Toppings: optional, see links in blog post for recipes
- guacamole
- pico de gallo
- poached egg

Instructions

- Note: The ground turkey I buy is the consistency of hamburger. If yours seems to have extra liquid, set on paper towels to drain juices.
- Place turkey, herbs, spices and lime in bowl and use hands to mix well.
- Form into four patties.
- Place pan on medium heat.
- Add olive oil to bottom of pan.
- When pan is hot, place patties in pan and cook for about 5 minutes each side or until cooked through.
- Top with guacamole, pico de gallo and poached egg if desired!

Ingredients

- 1 pound ground turkey, I prefer 85% lean, it has more fat which makes for a better burger!

If your ground turkey has excess liquid, be sure to set on paper towels to remove the juices.

- 1/2-3/4 of one jalapeño pepper, minced (I like it hot so I use 3/4)
- 1 medium size shallot, peeled and minced
- zest of one lime
- 2 Tablespoons chopped cilantro
- 1 teaspoon paprika
- 1 teaspoon cumin
- 1/2 a teaspoon sea salt
- 1/2 teaspoon black pepper
- Toppings: optional, see links in blog post for recipes
- guacamole
- pico de gallo
- poached egg

Instructions

- Note: The ground turkey I buy is the consistency of hamburger. If yours seems to have extra liquid, set on paper towels to drain juices.

- Place turkey, herbs, spices and lime in bowl and use hands to mix well.

- Form into four patties.

- Place pan on medium heat.

- Add olive oil to bottom of pan.

- When pan is hot, place patties in pan and cook for about 5 minutes each side or until cooked through.

- Top with guacamole, pico de gallo and poached egg if desired!

13. **Mexican Cauliflower Fried Rice**

Ingredients

- 12 oz riced cauliflower about 1 head, just shy of 4 cups
- 1 lb ground beef turkey, chicken, or pork
- 3 Tbsp cooking fat coconut oil, bacon fat, olive oil, ghee, divided
- 1/2 tsp fine grain sea salt
- 1/2 tsp onion powder
- 1/2 tsp garlic powder
- 1 tsp cumin
- 1 tsp chili powder
- generous dash chipotle pepper adjust to your taste or omit
- 1 red bell pepper diced
- 1 small yellow onion diced
- 3 garlic cloves minced
- 1 can chopped green chilis

- 1 jalapeno pepper seeds removed and minced

- Cilantro for garnish

- 1/2 cup homemade chipotle ranch dip

- 1 batch easy guac see below:

easy guac:

- 1 large ripe avocado or 2 small, mashed

- 2-3 Tbsp onion minced

- 1 clove garlic minced

- 1-2 Tbsp jalapeno peppers minced

- 1 1/2 Tbsp fresh lime juice

- 2 Tbsp chopped fresh cilantro plus more for garnish

Instructions

- Prepare the chipotle ranch, cover and chill until ready to serve.

- Heat a skillet over medium heat and add 1 Tbsp coconut oil.

- Add ground meat to skillet and sprinkle with salt and spices. Once browned, add onion, pepper and stir, cook about 45 seconds until softened.

- Add chopped green chilis, garlic, and jalapeno pepper and continue to cook another 45 seconds to heat through. Add cauli rice and stir to coat, then cover skillet for 30 seconds to soften cauliflower, remove from heat.

- Before serving, mash together all the guac ingredients in a bowl. To serve fried rice, top with extra cilantro, chipotle ranch and guac. Enjoy!

14. **Paleo Roasted Brussels Sprouts with Bacon & Apples**

Ingredients

- 1 lb brussels sprouts washed, tops removed and cut in half
- 2 tsp olive oil + sea salt to taste for roasting
- 1 medium pink lady apple {or other tart/sweet crisp apple}
- 4-6 slices nitrate free bacon sugar free (for Whole30)
- 1 Tbsp fresh rosemary finely chopped
- additional salt and pepper to taste

Instructions

- For this recipe you will roast your brussels sprouts while cooking the bacon and apples in a skillet on the stovetop.
- Preheat your oven to 400 degrees and line a large baking sheet with parchment paper. Make sure the brussels sprouts halves are uniform in size, if not, cut the larger pieces to ensure even cooking. Toss them with the 2 tsp

olive oil + salt and spread out on a parchment lined baking sheet. Roast them in the preheated oven for about 20 minutes, until they're browning and fork tender.

- Core the apple and chop into 1/2-1 inch cubes, set aside.

- Heat a medium heavy skillet over med-hi heat (I love my cast iron for this!) and cut your bacon into one inch pieces (my favorite knife does a great job with this)
- Add the bacon to the skillet and cook, stirring until about 3/4 of the way done (according to your own preference). At this point, add the apples and chopped rosemary and continue to cook and stir until the apples have softened and the bacon is fully cooked, adjusting the heat to avoid excessive browning if necessary. Remove from heat.

- Once brussels sprouts are done, add them to the skillet and toss to combine all the flavors. Sprinkle with more salt and pepper, if desire, and serve hot! This can be served as a side dish or with fried eggs for breakfast. Enjoy!

15. Turkish Stuffed Eggplant (Imam Bayildi)

Ingredients

- 1/2 cup extra-virgin olive oil
- 4 small eggplant (about 1 lb. 12 oz.)
- Kosher salt
- 2 cups minced leek (about 1 medium, rinsed, dark green leaves removed)
- 1 cup diced green bell pepper (about 1 medium, stem, seeds, and pith removed)
- 1/2 cup minced cauliflower
- 4 minced garlic cloves

- 3 1/2 cups grated Roma tomato, excess liquid drained (about 2 lb. or 13 medium tomatoes)
- 1/2 cup minced parsley
- 2 tbsp. minced fresh oregano
- 1 1/2 tbsp. maras pepper
- 1 cup crumbled feta or shanklish cheese (5 oz.)

Instructions

- Preheat oven to 375°and line a sheet tray with well-oiled parchment paper. Slice each eggplant in half lengthwise and brush them generously, all over, with olive oil. Season with kosher salt and place the halves, cut side down, on the prepared tray. Roast the eggplant until it is just starting to collapse and is tender when poked with a fork, about 25 minutes.
- Meanwhile, heat 2 tablespoons of olive oil over medium-high heat. Add the leek and sauté until soft but not yet browned, 5–6 minutes. Add

the bell pepper, cauliflower, and garlic, and continue cooking 5–8 minutes more, until the vegetables are tender and fragrant. Remove the vegetable mixture from the heat and stir in the freshly grated tomatoes and herbs. Season to taste with mara pepper and kosher salt.

- When the eggplant is cool enough to handle, use a thin spatula to peel the halves gently away from the parchment. Flip them over and smother them with as much of the vegetable mixture as possible (about 1⁄2 cup per half). Drizzle with the remaining 2 tablespoons of olive oil and return the pan to the oven for 10 minutes, or until the eggplant is hot and sizzly.

- Carefully transfer the eggplant to a large platter and garnish with crumbled feta or shanklish cheese before serving.

16. **Chocolate Dipped Frozen Bananas**

Ingredients

- 12 ounces dark chocolate, melted over a double boiler with 1 tablespoon coconut oil

- 3 large bananas, cut into thirds

- popsicle sticks

- chopped salted pistachios

- chopped spiced or smoked almonds

- cocoa nibs

- Melt chocolate over a double boiler (or in the microwave, if you prefer) with coconut oil. Stir until smooth, glossy, and entirely melted.

- Insert a popsicle stick into one end of each banana piece. Dip each banana into the warm melted chocolate. Shake off excess chocolate as best you can. Place dipped bananas on a parchment lined baking sheet. Sprinkle generously with chopped pistachios, chopped almonds, or cocoa nibs. Place in the freezer to harden and set.

- When frozen through wrap individually or enjoy immediately.

17. HOT CHOCOLATE WITH SUPERFOODS

Ingredients

- 2 cups non-dairy milk of choice (I used coconut but hemp or almond are great)
- 2 tbsp raw cacao (or cocoa powder)
- 1 tsp maca powder*
- 1/4 tsp ground turmeric
- 1/2 tsp of ground cinnamon
- 1 tbsp raw honey (or more to taste)
- 1 tbsp coconut oil

Instructions

- Add milk of choice to a medium-sized sauce pot and bring to a boil.
- Lower to a simmer and add cacao powder and stir.
- Add in maca powder, turmeric and cinnamon and continue to stir.
- Stir in honey until well combined.
- Add coconut oil and whip in until all chunks are melted and mixture becomes thick.
- Serve immediately.

18. Grain Free Blueberry Coffee Cake

Ingredients

Cake:

- ¼ cup honey
- ¼ cup butter or coconut oil (Paleo option), melted

- 4 eggs
- ½ cup almond milk
- ¾ cup almond flour
- ½ cup + 1 Tbsp coconut flour
- 2 tsp baking powder
- ½ tsp salt
- 1 Cup Blueberries

Streusel:

- 1 cup chopped pecans or walnuts
- 2 Tbsp honey
- ¼ cup butter or coconut oil
- 1½ tsp cinnamon
- 1 tsp coconut flour

Glaze:

- 2 Tbsp coconut butter, softened
- 1-2 Tbsp maple syrup
- ½ tsp salt

Instructions

- Preheat oven to 350 degrees

- Grease an 8x8 inch baking pan with butter or coconut oil.

- Combine almond flour, ½ cup coconut flour, baking powder and salt.

- In separate bowl combine honey, butter or coconut oil, eggs and almond milk.

- Mix wet ingredients into dry and and mix well.

- In a separate bowl mix together all streusel ingredients.

- In prepared baking pan place half of the cake dough and top with half of the streusel. Repeat.

- Top with 1 cup of blueberries.

- Bake for 30 minutes or until knife inserted comes out clean.

- Prepare glaze by mixing softened coconut butter and maple syrup.

- Spoon onto coffee cake and eat!

19. **Gluten-Free Vegan Chocolate Zucchini Bread**

Ingredients For Gluten-Free Chocolate Zucchini Bread

- 2 chia eggs (2 Tbsp ground chia or seeds + 6 Tbsp water)
- 1/3 cup unsweetened applesauce (or one single pack)
- One medium banana (about 1/2 cup)
- 1/3 cup sugar substitute (Splenda or baking stevia)
- 1 1/2 tsp baking soda
- 1 tsp baking powder
- 1/4 tsp salt
- 1/2 cup unsweetened cocoa powder
- 1/4 cup olive oil
- 1/4 cup unsweetened non-dairy milk*

- 1 cup grated zucchini or other squash (make sure to squeeze all the water out first)
- 3/4 cup gluten-free flour (I use the pre-made kind made by King Arthur or Bob's Red Mill.)
- 1/3 cup gluten-free oat flour
- 1/3 cup almond flour**

Optional add-ons or alternatives:
- 1/2 cup pecans or walnuts***
- Non-dairy chocolate chips
- Ground flax meal instead of ground chia or chia seeds
- (Nutrition facts below don't include info for the add-ons)

Unsweetened almond milk is a really good low-calorie, no-sugar choice. I also really like Oatley brand oat milk as a non-dairy liquid. But keep in mind that, while it doesn't have added sugar, oat milk does have natural carbs that you break down into sugar.

Almond flour, which is different than almond meal, helps with texture and adds protein and fiber. But it can be pricey. You might be able to double the oat flour or switch out gluten-free flour if you don't want to buy it. I've done that for other recipes, but not this one specifically. So experiment at your own risk.

I don't add extra walnuts or pecans to things with bananas or oat and almond flour. All of those ingredients are digestively ok for me to snack on by themselves. Each one has moderate amounts of FODMAPs — carbs that cause gas. When I mix the nuts into this zucchini bread, I always get a little more bloated than I'm comfortable with.

Directions

- Preheat the oven to 375 degrees. Spray a 9x5-inch loaf pan with some nonstick spray.

- Mix the chia eggs together and let sit for 5 minutes or so.

- In a big bowl, mix together the mashed banana, artificial sweetener, baking soda, baking powder, salt, and cocoa powder.

- Add the chia mix.

- Pour in the olive oil and non-dairy milk. Mix.

- Stir in the zucchini.

- Add the flours.

- If using chocolate chips, stir those in last.

- Put in the loaf pan and bake for 45 minutes.

- I cooked my bread for 45 minutes, but you may need to leave it in a little longer. Everyone's oven is a little different. You can stick a knife or toothpick in the middle to see if it's done. It should come out clean.

- Storage of the bread

I usually wait for a half-hour to an hour before I cut into it. You could probably dig in after it cools for 5 to 10 minutes. I store it in the fridge if I'm going to eat it fast. Otherwise, I'll slice it up into single servings and keep it in the freezer. The recipe makes about 10 good-size servings. However, you could make it 12 if you want smaller pieces.

I thaw out bread one of a few ways: naturally on the counter, in a toaster oven, or wrapped in a damp paper towel and zapped for 30 seconds or so in the microwave.

Enjoy!

20. **Spicy Lentil Soup**

Ingredients

- 2 tbs oil
- 1 onion, chopped
- 2 celery sticks, chopped
- 2 carrots, chopped
- Garlic - put in as much as you want - garlic has many health benefits
- 4oz red lentils, rinsed
- 1 pint vegetable stock
- Salt and pepper
- Curry powder

Directions

- In a pan, cook onion, carrot, and celery with a little oil till soft. Add remaining ingredients, bring to the boil and simmer for 45 minutes, stirring occasionally. If you are adding some ground spices, add them at the beginning and lightly fry them off - this will bring out the oils and increase the flavour.

- Check seasoning. Serve with a swirl of nut yogurt or plain yogurt and chopped coriander (cilantro) leaves